C000078983

How to Look
After Yourself
When You're
Feeling Depressed

How to Look After Yourself When You're Feeling Depressed

A Little Book of Encouragement

Alice Rosewell

THE CHOIR PRESS

Copyright © 2016 Alice Rosewell

All rights reserved. No part of this publication may be reproduced or transmitted in any form or by any means, electronic or mechanical including photocopying, recording or any information storage or retrieval system, without prior permission in writing from the publishers.

The right of Alice Rosewell to be identified as the author of this work has been asserted by her in accordance with the Copyright, Designs and Patents Act 1988

Illustrations by LCG Design

First published in the United Kingdom in 2016 by
The Choir Press

ISBN 978-1-910864-53-1

Also by Alice Rosewell:

Fleur and Jane
A story of friendship and secrets, available on
Amazon Kindle.

Contents

Preface

One Friday evening, I went to bed after a hard week doing a job I wasn't enjoying, and looking forward to a weekend of relaxation and fun.

On the Saturday morning I woke up and found that overnight all the colour and pleasure had drained away from the world. Damn! Damn! Damn! Depression had found its way into my head again and was squatting there like a poisonous toad, robbing me of all energy and any desire to move. All I wanted to do was get back under the duvet and stay there until the Monday morning alarm forced me out of bed again.

What a waste of a weekend! I was annoyed. I imagined waking up on Monday with matted hair and no clean clothes to put on. What I needed was a kind person who could inject a little energy into my poor crushed mind and encourage me, at the very least, to get up and see if there was anything useful I could do, even if it was joyless hard work. Of course there was no one available; people without depression are out enjoying their weekends, dammit!

When you're depressed even making the decision to get out of bed can seem insurmountable. In fact, making the decision can be much harder than actually doing it. Only someone who has suffered from depression will understand this. So I decided to make all my decisions for the day while still in bed. I found some paper and a pencil, made a cup of tea (funny how easy that was!) and settled back into my project.

It worked for me that day, so I wrote down a plan that I could use for every day if I slipped into depression, and that was the start of this little book. This book is not designed as a cure for depression, or a way to achieve your goals; it's just some encouragement to keep going when the going is tough.

I hope it helps.

Introduction

Self-care is one of the things that can go by the board when we're depressed. It's SO much effort and it's SO pointless. Actually it's SO important. It keeps alive that fading flicker of self-esteem which is so important to recovery, and keeps your body healthy while you wait for the antidepressants to kick in, or the therapy or sports recovery plan to start delivering the goods, or simply for the black dog to bugger off and annoy someone else.

There are many routes to recovery for the determined depressive. Self-care on its own will not be sufficient to treat severe depression, but whatever state you're in, having someone take an interest in you and be kind to you will help, and where self-care is concerned, that someone has to be you.

What is depression?

There are clinical definitions for depression, and there are many books out there on the subject.

For the purposes of this little book I'm including everything from ennui – that feeling of boredom and 'can't be bothered' – through to the sort of depression that needs serious medical intervention.

Depression alters our behaviour in ways that are unhelpful and unwelcome to ourselves and other people. We may turn into slobs. We may reject our friends. We may become disengaged from our families. We may say or do things that lose us our jobs. We may neglect or even damage our health.

Depression impoverishes our lives.

When we are depressed we crave comfort, safety and escape. Escape from people who cause us emotional pain. Escape from fresh air which chills our fragile skin. Escape from noise and bright lights which assault our senses. If we dwell too long on these thoughts we can find ourselves longing for the ultimate escape and the safety to be found six feet under. But human beings are not supposed to be safe at any cost; we are supposed to live.

So stick two fingers up at the noonday demon that is depression, and resolve not to go down without a fight.

Who gets depression?

About one in four people in the UK, that's who!

Everybody gets the blues sometimes. Some people can shake it off, give themselves a good talking to and get on with things. These people can say, 'OK, not feeling too good right now, but tomorrow's another day!' People with depression say, 'Tomorrow's another day, and it'll be rubbish, just like this one.'

Rich, poor, old, young, clever, dim, single, married. There is no category immune to depression.

Why do we get depression?

This is a good question; working out why we're depressed could be the start of getting better.

Sometimes the reason is an irrevocable loss. There's no cure for this, only to breathe in, and breathe out, then do it again, and again.

It may be feeling trapped: in an unfulfilling job, a loveless marriage, caring for dependent parents.

It may be despair and helplessness: the wars and suffering in the world, our child's drug addiction.

Or there may be no identifiable reason, and in any case a reason is not a cure. Sometimes shit just happens.

One day at a time

I do like a good to-do list. Very often I can spend more time revising my lists, ordering, categorising, prioritising, than I do actually doing any of the tasks. Lists focus the mind and help you make decisions. Ticking items off the list makes you feel in control and gives a sense of satisfaction.

In the following pages I describe a series of self-care tasks which always make me feel better after (sometimes a long time after) I've done them. Some days I do most of them, some days I only manage one or two. The point is not to set a goal and then beat yourself up if you fall short. The point is to remind yourself of all the little ways you can look after yourself, and give yourself credit for every achievement.

The best days are the ones where I float through the first few tasks without even thinking. This is called 'not being depressed'. I try to cherish these times no matter how fleeting, not write them off as aberrations.

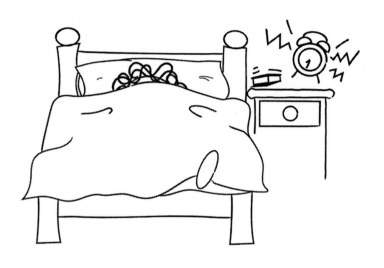

TASK 1
Wake up when the alarm goes off

Are you one of the many who press the snooze button every morning, sometimes not even registering that the alarm has sounded? You are not alone. Many people love their snooze button, but it is not your friend. You think that your need for an extra ten minutes' sleep outweighs all other considerations, and anyway another ten minutes is not going to hurt. Oh, but it does, it does! Some people plan to press the snooze button once, twice or three times before properly waking up, but why would you deliberately give yourself a half-hour of disturbed sleep before waking instead of setting the alarm for half an hour later?

Even if you haven't got a job to go to, make sure you set your alarm as if you did, and get yourself a whole day's worth of life – because you're worth it!

So, back to the alarm. Resist that snooze button – every ten minutes' snooze is ten minutes stolen from your morning routine, and that results in sick-making activities like rushing breakfast, not having time to make your lunch, and starting the day stressed. This is so horrible I'm feeling stressed just writing about it.

Easier said than done, you may say. Here's a way:

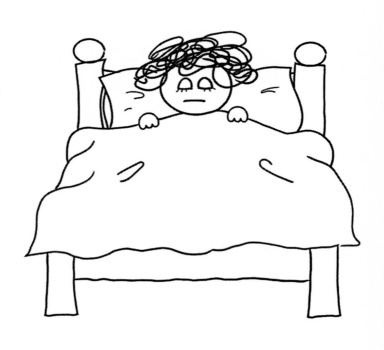

TASK 2
Sit up

Groan out loud if it helps. Swear, moan, complain, but get yourself upright. You don't have to open your eyes, you don't have to turn the light on. Wrap yourself in your dressing gown if it's cold; just make sure your face is uncovered, and start to breathe. Stretch your legs out in front of you and wiggle your toes. It's surprising how even the smallest stretch starts to wake the brain up.

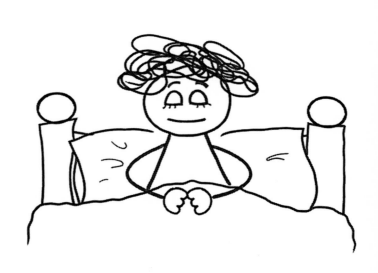

TASK 3
Meditate for five minutes

Everyone who knows anything knows that meditation is good for you, but most of us just never make the time. How mad is that? Remember that snooze button you didn't press? Well, here's a much better use of five minutes. And while five minutes may not be as good as twenty, it's infinitely better than nothing, and if you listen to Ruby Wax, who knows what she's talking about, sprinkling your day with moments of mindfulness can make all the difference to your mental wellbeing.

The crucial thing about meditation is that it is NOT an opportunity to ruminate on all the things that are wrong with your life. Every negative thought you experience during the day has to be processed and made sense of when you sleep. No wonder we often have trouble sleeping and wake up exhausted. If you can't stop your mind from racing, try focusing on relaxing your face, imagine those frown lines smoothing away, and breathe slowly.

There are lots of different ways to meditate. Some people use guided meditation CDs; my favourite is TM (transcendental meditation). So here's a project for you once you're getting a really good night's sleep: find the meditation technique that suits you.

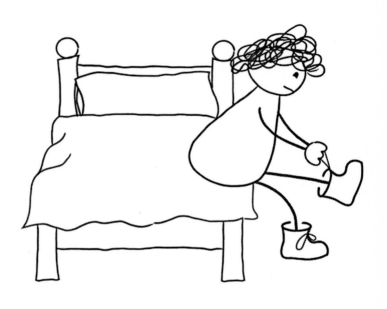

TASK 4
Get up

OK, this is it, the big heave! What can you do to make this less daunting? Music to get the blood pumping, some cosy slippers for cold mornings. Once you're on your feet, reach up and stretch, then reach down and touch your toes (or knees – whatever you can manage). Do this three times. It's an old-fashioned exercise, but surprisingly effective.

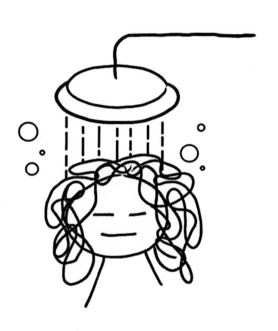

TASK 5
Go to the bathroom

This shouldn't be too difficult. Your bladder probably wants to go even if your brain doesn't yet.

Here's where the first major piece of self-care happens. Get naked! This is one of the things that goes by the wayside when we get depressed. Even the thought of washing can be exhausting, but it's *so* worth the effort. Showers are good, but if you don't have the energy, go retro; an all-over wash with a flannel is fine. Just wash away the sweat and smells. I guarantee you won't feel worse and will probably feel a smidge better.

And another project: make your bathroom a place you feel good in. Clean and tidy is a good start and doesn't cost much. Do you have a plant to talk to in the morning? Pick one that has air cleaning properties, like the peace lily. Can you splash out on some colourful towels – or some luxury soap?

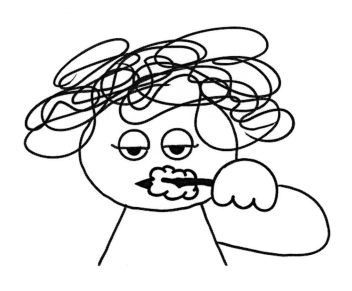

TASK 6
Clean your teeth

Oh, the minty freshness! Who could fail to be uplifted? But there are much more important reasons to get your teeth clean than just getting rid of that 'bottom of a parrot's cage' taste. Having your teeth drilled is unpleasant enough, but gum disease is far more dangerous. Apart from the risk of gingivitis and losing all your teeth in one go, inflamed gums give bacteria an easy route into your system and can cause a whole host of other illnesses up to and including heart disease. So break open that piggy bank and invest in a good electric toothbrush and some of those little interdental brushes. Now, if you ever feel like smiling, you won't have to worry about halitosis or the state of your teeth.

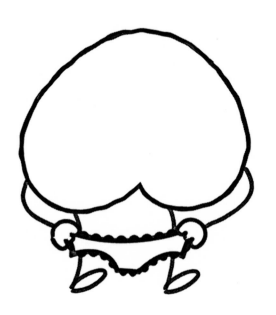

TASK 7
Get dressed

Clean underwear, please! And not just because you might get knocked down and taken to hospital. Wearing the same knickers/boxers all day, all night, and the next day registers very high on most people's yuckometer and, let's face it, if you're depressed you already have enough yuck in your life. New pants (underpants to you Americans) are not expensive, and give you a little nudge up the self-esteem ladder. Most of the girls I know think that nice new undies are a tonic, and I have it on good authority that the guys feel the same.

If you've sorted out your clothes the night before (fast-forward to task 22), they should all be laid out ready to put on – so no decisions to make and no stress there.

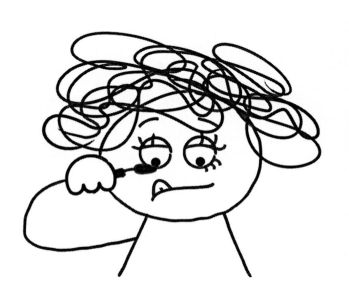

TASK 8
Fix your hair and make-up

Vanity, vanity, we have it for a reason. People who take care of their appearance (men and women) are taken more seriously by others, and who doesn't love a bit of respect? I'm not talking about fake tan and inch-long eyelashes, although I know that's a minimum standard for some. I'm saying, when you look in the mirror do you say, 'Yep, happy with that. I'm good to go,' or do you spend the day trying to avoid mirrors and making excuses for letting yourself go?

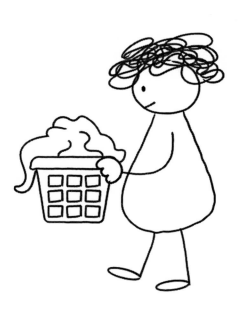

TASK 9
Clear your bedroom

There is no doubt that the quality of your bedroom affects the quality of your sleep. You don't need new furniture and carpets to make a difference. Once again, clean and tidy will improve your mood, so take a couple of minutes to throw back the bedcovers and let the air in, then clear away all your dirty laundry, crockery and any other rubbish. If you're still living at home with parents this will earn you serious brownie points.

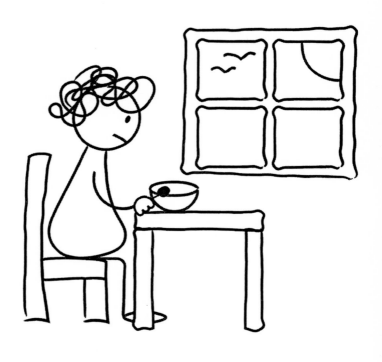

TASK 10
Have breakfast

The most important meal of the day, we are told. Whatever yours is – full English, healthy yoghurt and fruit, or coffee and an aspirin – take time to sit near a window and look out while you're eating. Let your mind roam free for a few minutes; let it escape from your own four walls, whether it's pottering around your garden or nosing into the window of the opposite flat. This can be difficult if you're a parent, I know, especially if you've got a screaming toddler hanging around your neck. Could it be worth getting up a bit earlier to avoid indigestion?

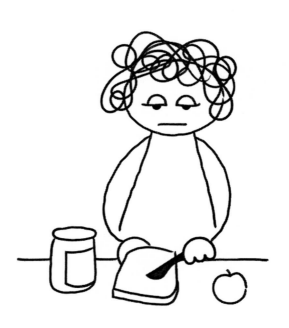

TASK 11
Make your packed lunch

Few of us are fortunate enough to have a work canteen, or a handy bistro where we can get a good lunch. The alternatives are often pretty grim: chips, sandwiches full of fat and salt, fizzy drinks, sugary desserts and pastries, and caffeine. They fill us up and satisfy the reward centres in our brains at least for a while, but we usually pay for it with an energy crash in the afternoon, not to mention the damage to our purses and wallets.

Getting into the habit of making your own lunch is going to save you money in the short term, and if financial stress is one of the things getting you down that's got to be a good thing. Once you have the habit, you may want to start tinkering with the menu to introduce more mind-healthy options – out with the cakes, and in with the crudités – although this might take a bit of working up to.

Even if you don't go out to work you may want to do this, or just write down what you're going to eat during the day. This will give you an aspirational eating routine and serve as a reminder not to pick mindlessly at whatever is most convenient.

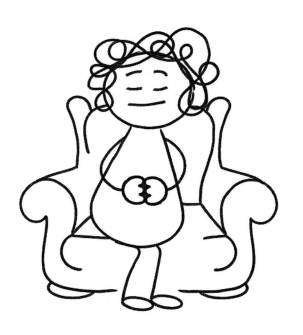

TASK 12
Meditate for fifteen minutes

So, you're all clean, shiny and fed, and if you got your act together you now have fifteen minutes to meditate. Resist the temptation to get to work early and start on that email backlog – this is more important. If your time has got away from you again, try sitting down and taking three long, slow breaths. Find your centre, if you know where it is, and make sure you don't leave the house primed for an accident or argument.

If it's a cold day, put your slippers on the radiator before you go out; you'll be glad of them later.

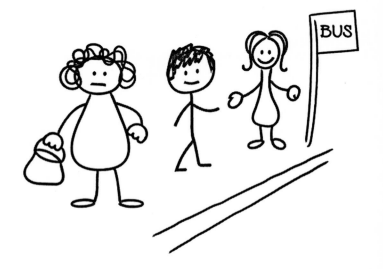

TASK 13
Go to work

Firstly, for people who go out to work, try to travel at the least stressful time you can manage. If your organisation offers flexible working hours, try to avoid the rush hour; this will save time and stress. If possible, incorporate some walking into your commute, even if that only means parking at the farthest end of the car park.

Once you're at work, do the best you can. When you're depressed just getting to work is an achievement, so don't be too hard on yourself. On the other hand, laziness and self-pity are forms of self-harm; avoid them. And then there are the people, some good and supportive, and some mean and destructive. Focus on the good and shrug off the bad if possible. Remember, happy people are not mean and rude, so the bad guys could be suffering as much as you are.

Secondly, for people not working, or working from home, go out anyway. Take a walk around the block and mull over what you're going to do with your day. The television is your enemy here, so don't even think about spending your day on the couch. You could do something lucrative, like setting up your own business or searching for a job, or worthy, like editing the parish newsletter, or personally fulfilling, like knitting, baking, doing a jigsaw puzzle; just make it more mean-ingful than watching daytime TV or lying in bed crying.

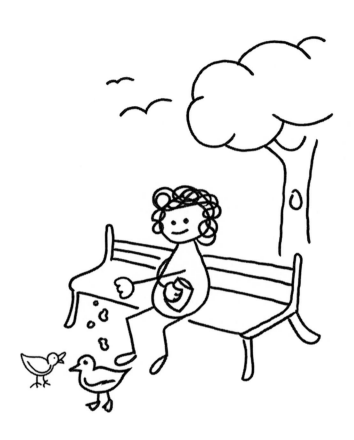

TASK 14
Take a proper lunch break

Hah, made it to lunch time. Give yourself a pat on the back, and a proper lunch break. Most of us who work in offices find that the management are quite happy for us to work through the lunch hours, dropping crumbs into our keyboards. Don't let them get away with it! Your health demands and deserves some time away from your desk. Get out of the building if you can and take a brisk walk. Rustle up some workmates to take your lunch outside or, at the very least, go and visit someone else's desk and make sure they turn their monitor off for an hour while you eat.

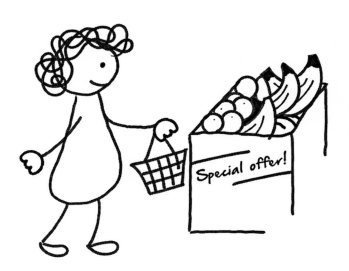

TASK 15
Go food shopping on the way home

The end of the day and you want to get home so badly you want to cry. The thought of shopping makes you feel sick and faint, but hang in there. No matter how high your anxiety, there's a pretty good chance you won't collapse into the broccoli display. Breathe slowly, walk slowly; you're in doctor mode now, and you need to look after the poor sick patient that is your poor depressed self. 'Let food be thy medicine,' Hippocrates is supposed to have said. There are plenty of books, YouTube videos and internet articles on what diet is best for you, but when it comes to depression, more veg and less sugar is a good place to start.

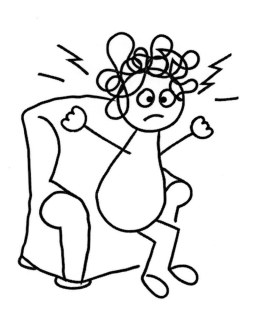

TASK 16
Don't sit down yet!

How many times have you walked in the door at the end of the day, dumped your bags, sat down with your coat still on, and stared at the wall for an hour? Been there, done that. Sometimes it feels like there's not the tiniest drop of energy left, and you just sit until you feel it's late enough to go to bed (7.30?) and you drag yourself upstairs.

If you can possibly manage it, don't sit down when you get home. Switch to auto-pilot and do the following:

1. Change out of your work clothes. If it's a cold day and you've completed task 12, your warm slippers will be a delight.
2. Prepare the veg you'll need for your dinner.
3. Put away your groceries.
4. Put the kettle on.

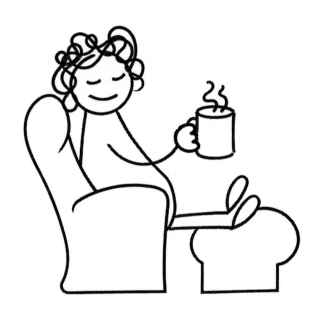

TASK 17
Have a cup of tea and a sit down

Make yourself a cup of tea or drink of your choice – no, not a G&T or bottle of beer; we all know where that leads, and we're trying to be mindful, remember? Put your feet up. Relax. Celebrate the fact you've got through another day and give yourself credit for every effort you've made, no matter how small.

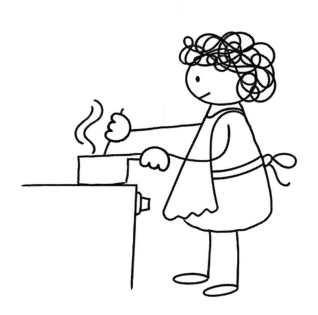

TASK 18
Make dinner

The effort of cooking often feels like too much at the end of the day; even if your depression has left you some appetite, a fish finger sandwich or a tin of soup may seem the most you can manage. That's better than nothing, but if you've succeeded in preparing your veg earlier it'll be much easier to fling it all in a steamer now and treat your body to some real nutrition, not to mention fibre. A bunged-up gut can make even the most cheerful person miserable, so you don't want to add that to your troubles.

At the other end of the scale, food, especially junk, may be your consolation of choice, and your ideal evening may be gorging on takeaways and ice cream until you explode. Plan ahead if you think your diet is not doing you any good, and make sure you get the nutrition in before any junk.

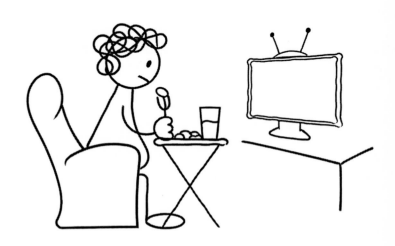

TASK 19
Eat dinner

The best option for eating dinner is sitting at a table with convivial friends and maybe a glass of wine. If that only happens once a year on Christmas Day, you may have to make do with your own company. Now is the time when television might be your friend. Sharing your dinner with Sherlock or Dr Brian Cox can be a real pleasure. Just remember to eat slowly and taste your food – you might find you like it.

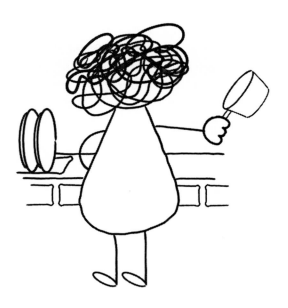

TASK 20
Wash up

If you read *Zen and the Art of Motorcycle Maintenance*, you will discover that washing up can have its own intrinsic pleasure. For most people suffering from depression this might be a bit of a stretch. The rewards of a clean kitchen are felt later, when you can find a clean saucepan to make your evening cocoa, and even more when you stagger into the kitchen in the morning and are faced with a sink completely empty of dirty dishes.

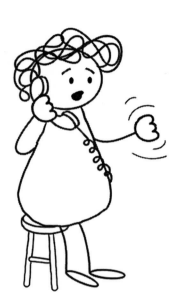

TASK 21
Phone a friend

Every book on recovering from depression will extol the value of connecting with family and friends. You may feel that you have become a burden to everyone who knows you, and every call that goes to voicemail, or email that fails to get a response, just convinces you more that people are avoiding you. Persevere. People like to help. Just try not to drone on about your depression unless you're sure the person listening gets it. Until you're feeling better, try to avoid:

- People who freak out and think depressed equals suicidal; you'll end up having to reassure them.
- People who tell you that you have lots to be grateful and happy about. You know that already. Depression is an illness, not a lack of shoes/boyfriend/perfect teeth/youth ...
- People who want to fix you and have just heard about a marvellous new 'cure' for depression which involves eating only beetroot for a month or some such.
- People who know someone else who's been depressed but SOOO much worse than you, and then talk at length about someone you've never met and wouldn't be interested in if you had.

You may think 'who does that leave?' Well, if you're lucky you have a friend who will be happy to talk gloom for a few minutes and then turn the conversation to more upbeat topics. If not, restrict the subject matter to gossip and plans for the weekend. And try to forgive the people who don't get it. They may love you very much but find the whole subject of mental illness bewildering or even frightening, like parenthood or bereavement.

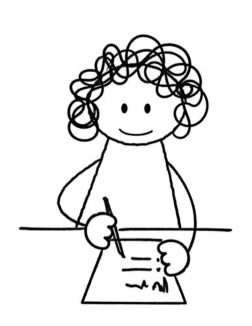

TASK 22
Plan for tomorrow

Here's where you set yourself up for success tomorrow, even if today has been a bit of a wash-out. Go through all the tasks in this little book and make sure you've prepared in advance everything you can that will make it easier for you to look after yourself.

- Are you running out of toothpaste? Start your shopping list.

- What are you going to eat for dinner tomorrow? If it's not in the house, put it on the list.

- What are going to wear tomorrow? Lay your clothes out before you go to bed.

- Can't get it together to make lunch in the morning? Do it now.

- And so on ...

Give yourself a head start so you don't have to make any decisions first thing in the morning.

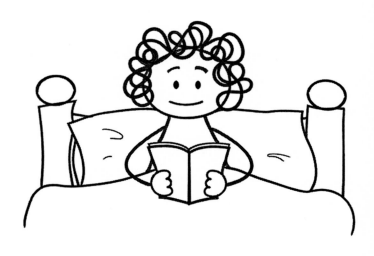

TASK 23
Go to bed with a good book

An uplifting or cheerful book is my way of getting in the mood for sleep. You might sleep better after listening to whale song on CD, or soaking in a hot bath. Just avoid screens, especially the sort which emit a lot of blue light (laptops, some phones), as these have been proven to mess with your body clock and may stop you getting to sleep for hours.

If you are regularly in a very deep sleep when the alarm goes off, you may not be getting enough or the right kind of sleep. Experiment with your diet, hot milk at bedtime, bedsocks to keep your feet warm, and if you have the means, check out the various sleep apps you can download onto your phone. When I first started monitoring my sleep, I was amazed how restless I was. The answer for me was not eating starch in the evening (weird?); for you it might be reading a chapter of an uplifting book, or a relaxing yoga routine before bed. Finding the right sleep hygiene routine is a little project which will reap benefits whether you're sick or well.

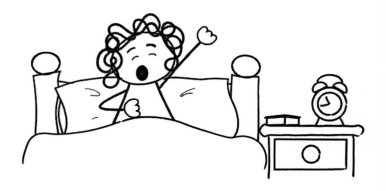

TASK 24
Set alarm and turn the light off

So here we are at the end of the day. Hopefully you can look back and say that you are satisfied with what you've achieved, but even if you haven't done a single thing on the list, don't beat yourself up.

Remember we're not trying for a cure for depression here; there are experts for that. We're just trying to keep it together so that one day, when the sun comes out again, we'll be fit and healthy enough to enjoy it.

What next?

I hope you recognised some of the situations in the last chapter. Of course, depending on your situation, your self-care needs might be quite different. For instance, you may be a student living independently for the first time, or retired and caring for elderly parents.

Try and write down your own self-care needs. Remember, this is not a wishlist; it's the things that will make you feel a little better and a lot more in control if you do them on a daily basis.

Don't underestimate how hard self-care is when you're depressed, and make sure your list is something that motivates you, not a stick to beat yourself with.

High days and holidays

Getting through the week can be tough when you're depressed, but at least there's the weekend to look forward to.

Alas! At weekends and holidays it's sometimes even harder to keep the blues at bay. We look forward to our days off, we have expectations of fun, enjoyment, happiness; and the disappointment when these fail to materialise is all the worse if they have been keenly anticipated.

But why should we be surprised? The whole thing about depression is that it sucks all the pleasure and feeling of purpose out of life, regardless of the day of the week.

What to do?

You can try to escape from the depression, stay in bed all day, or medicate yourself with alcohol, drugs or food. The lure of oblivion is so tempting. In the moment these options seem like a good idea, and may give some temporary relief from the mental pain, but be honest: how long does that feeling last? Five minutes, an hour, an evening? And in the aftermath do you beat yourself up for wasting another day?

Denial is an option. 'Depressed? Me? No, no, no, just a bit tired!' and you can fake your way through the weekend pretending to yourself and everyone else that nothing is wrong, and suffering even more exhaustion as a result of all that emotional effort trying to keep that sunny smile from slipping.

Neither of those options will do you any good, and days off are too precious to be thrown away. It's not possible to find peace of mind by frantically searching, but it is possible to make an environment where peace and even happiness might show up unexpectedly.

Remember that weekends are not the time when your real life happens. Every day is your real life. Weekends are supposed to be the time when you rest after the week's work and recharge your batteries for the next week.

Planning and mindfulness are the key. Think ahead and schedule some activities which you will feel good about doing, without depending on some immediate gratification. A walk in the country, a trip to the cinema, even some long-put-off chores like putting up a picture or cleaning out the shower trap. There may be spells of contentment, satisfaction, or even cheerfulness. Enjoy them, but don't try to hang on to them. Trust that others will come in their own time.

Most importantly, make sure you've allowed time for rest. Not lying on the sofa with a box set and a pint of ice cream, although this certainly has a place in a healthy lifestyle, but real rest – dozing in the garden for a couple of hours, or listening to relaxing music: anything that allows you to close your eyes, let your body be still and calm your mind. No doubt you will experience negative thoughts, but try to separate them from present reality. Imagine them drifting away on the breeze. Can you see yourself not suffering, just being relaxed and content in the moment?

Inspiring people, inspiring words

In your lowest moments you may think that life is pointless, maybe you feel that the best years are behind you, maybe you can see nothing ahead but grey drudgery. When you're depressed you just can't see any light at the end of the tunnel.

But think of the great and good who have trudged this doleful path before you, still leading interesting, useful and even spectacular lives despite periods of black depression. For instance:

JK Rowling, author of the *Harry Potter* stories, who said:

> Depression is the most unpleasant thing I have ever experienced ... It is that absence of being able to envisage that you will ever be cheerful again. The absence of hope. That very deadened feeling, which is so very different from feeling sad. Sad hurts but it's a healthy feeling. It is a necessary thing to feel. Depression is very different.
>
> *JK Rowling speaking to Ann Treneman, 'Harry and me', The Times,*
> *30 June 2000*

Winston Churchill, politician and wartime UK prime minister, also painted watercolours which are now prized by collectors, and wrote the definitive history of Britain. He referred to his depression as 'the black dog', and wrote:

> I don't like standing near the edge of a platform when an express train is passing through. I like to stand right back and if possible get a pillar between me and the train. I don't like to stand by the side of a ship and look down into the water. A second's action would end everything. A few drops of desperation.

Some have written words that can bring comfort or at least the reassurance that you are understood by an army of fellow sufferers and supporters. For example:

> Listen to the people who love you. Believe that they are worth living for even when you don't believe it. Seek out the memories depression takes away and project them into the future. Be brave; be strong; take your pills. Exercise because it's good for you even if every step weighs a thousand pounds. Eat when food itself disgusts you. Reason with yourself when you have lost your reason.
>
> *Andrew Solomon, The Noonday Demon:*
> *An Atlas of Depression, 2001*

> Every man has his secret sorrows which the world knows not; and often times we call a man cold when he is only sad.
> *Henry Wadsworth Longfellow, Hyperion, 1839*

> 'The best thing for being sad,' replied Merlin ... 'is to learn something. That's the only thing that never fails. You may grow old and trembling in your anatomies, you may lie awake at night listening to the disorder of your veins, you may miss your only love, you may see the world about you devastated by evil lunatics, or know your honour trampled in the sewers of baser minds. There is only one thing for it then – to learn. Learn why the world wags and what wags it. That is the only thing which the mind can never exhaust, never alienate, never be tortured by, never fear or distrust, and never dream of regretting. Learning is the only thing for you. Look what a lot of things there are to learn.'
> *TH White, The Once and Future King, 1958*

Try keeping a notebook in your bag or pocket and jot down any insights you have into your own state of mind. There may be patterns you're not yet aware of, helpful or unhelpful activities, mind-healthy recipes or uplifting poems. No rambling on about how bad you feel, though; you know that already. This should be your own little book of encouragement, tailored just for you.

Whoever you are and whatever you have done with your life so far, the world is full of compassionate people who want you to be well and happy.

Be one of them!

Further reading

Here are some books that I've found useful:

Sod It! The Depression 'Virus' and How to Deal With It,
Martin Davies, Talking Life, 2006

Funny, insightful and instructive. A really useful book for anyone who is depressed or knows someone who is. And if you don't have the energy to read the words, you can colour in the pictures.

Mind over Mood: Change How You Feel by Changing the Way You Think, Dennis Greenberger and Christine Padesky, Guilford Press, 1995

If you've made the commitment to take responsibility for your recovery, this workbook will help show you the way. It really helped me understand how my own thinking habits were setting the scene for depression, and what I could do about it.

Human Givens: The New Approach to Emotional Health and Clear Thinking, Joe Griffin and Ivan Tyrrell, HG Publishing, 2013

This is a dauntingly large book; however, if you're interested in some of the latest thinking on emotional health, it's an intriguing read. If you don't have the strength to tackle the whole book, the chapter on depression gives much food for thought, particularly the interrelation between depression and unhealthy sleep patterns.

Zen and the Art of Motorcycle Maintenance, Robert M Pirsig, Vintage, 1991

Uplifting and thought-provoking. A classic.

Sane New World: Taming the Mind, Ruby Wax, Hodder, 2014

If you're of a scientific turn of mind you'll love Ruby's descriptions of what's going on in the depressed brain. Even if you're not, her explanation of the value of mindfulness is very illuminating and motivating. And funny? I tittered all the way through!

Eat & Run: My Unlikely Journey to Ultramarathon Greatness, Scott Jurek, Bloomsbury, 2013

What sort of mind allows a body to run a hundred miles? This is an amazing insight into the 'just do it' approach to life. Not preachy, no 'if you want it badly enough' magical thinking nonsense. Just find your support group, learn what you have to do, and do it!

Lightning Source UK Ltd.
Milton Keynes UK
UKOW01f1719090616

275934UK00024B/1/P